Endometriosis Diet
Heal Naturally With Nutritional Therapy

Barbara Williams

Copyright © dsk-enterprise Inc., 2015

All rights reserved. No part of this publication may be reproduced in any form without written consent of the author and the publisher. The information contained in this book may not be stored in a retrieval system, or transmitted in any form by any means, electronic, mechanical, photocopying or otherwise without the written consent of the publisher. This book may not be resold, hired out or otherwise disposed by way of trade in any form of binding or cover other than that in which it is published, without the written consent of the publisher. Respective authors own all copyrights not held by the publisher. The presentation of the information is without contract or any type of guarantee assurance. All trademarks and brands within this book are for clarifying purposes only and are the owned by the owners themselves, not affiliated with this document.

Legal Disclaimer

The information contained in this book is strictly for educational purpose only. The content of this book is the sole expression and opinion of its author and not necessarily that of the publisher. It is not intended to cure, treat, and diagnose any kind of disease or medical condition. It is sold with the understanding that the publisher is not rendering any type of medical, psychological, legal, or any other kind of professional advice. You should seek the services of a competent professional before applying concepts in this book. Neither the publisher nor the individual author(s) shall be liable for any physical, psychological, emotional, financial, or commercial damages, directly or indirectly by the use of this material, which is provided "as is", and without warranties. Therefore, if you wish to apply ideas contained in this book, you are taking full responsibility for your actions.

Table of Contents

1: What is Endometriosis?

2: Signs and Symptoms and How to Control Them

3: Nutritional Therapy for Treating Endometriosis

4: Foods You Should Take

5: Foods That You Should Avoid

6: Natural Treatments and Therapy for Healing Endometriosis

7: Exercise and Endometriosis

8: Adopt Dietary and Lifestyle Changes to Manage Endometriosis

Conclusion

Introduction

Have you been diagnosed with endometriosis? This is a practical book with the most effective nutritional therapy that you will find helpful in healing Endometriosis. The dietary approach strengthens the immune system to help it fight diseases and as a result, endometriosis symptoms are alleviated.

You don't have to look so far, many of the things you need may be right there on your kitchen shelf. This book will be of great help to you if you want to overcome the signs and symptoms of Endometriosis. If you have not been diagnosed with Endometriosis, you will still gain a lot by applying the natural approach recommended, to prevent this disease.

A healthy diet and nutrition are essential not only for those suffering from endometriosis but for your overall health. I am sure that, the natural healthy diet offered in this "must-read" book will help you heal naturally and regain your vibrant health again.

1: What is Endometriosis?

Endometriosis is a chronic disease that affects women and girls. The endometriosis tissue normally lines up the uterine cavity and is known as endometrium. When endometriosis tissue grows outside the uterus, it may develop in the ovaries, fallopian tubes and elsewhere. It causes pain, heavy periods, spotting or excessive bleeding between periods and infertility among other symptoms.

Endometrial tissue that has grown outside the uterus has similarity to endometrium in the uterus. Naturally, estrogen hormone is circulated in the body and it causes growth in the lining of the uterus which is shed off during the monthly periods when the eggs are not fertilized.

This is the same way that the flow of estrogen causes growth of endometrial tissue that has grown outside the uterus and when it is shed off, since it is not in its usual place within the uterus it aggravates the pain, cramps and bleeding experienced during the woman's monthly periods and at other times. As a result, spotting and heavy bleeding may occur between periods making the sufferer's life hectic.

There is hope for every sufferer in the nutritional therapy offered in this book.

Parts of the body affected by endometriosis

Endometriosis affects the:

- Ovaries
- Fallopian tubes
- Urinary bladder and/or ureters
- Cervix
- Back and front of the uterus as well as the outer surface of the uterus
- Uterine ligaments
- The abdominal cavity
- Intestines

The condition causes pelvic pain, cramps, heavy and irregular periods, infertility and other symptoms. It may also spread to the incision scars left after surgery. Women who have undergone abdominal surgery, cesarean section, laparoscopy, hysterectomy, appendectomy, ectopic pregnancies and hernia repair are pre-disposed to scar endometriosis.

Diagnosis of endometriosis

The health care provider observing the patient may suspect endometriosis as a result of physical examination, along with symptoms reported and the patient's health history. The endometrial tissue may be felt during pelvic examinations but pelvic ultrasound can be performed to confirm the diagnosis. Large endometriosis cysts can be visualized on the ultrasound but small ones cannot, so in such cases, other methods like laparoscopy may be used.

Laparoscopy technique uses cameras inserted through small abdominal incisions to visualize the endometrial tissue. At times when the lesions are not visible, biopsy may be used. Surgery can be used as a diagnosis or for the treatment of endometriosis.

Complications of endometriosis

Endometriosis can cause difficulty in the sufferer's ability to become pregnant and in some cases infertility can occur. In severe cases, it may cause some types of cancer.

- Infertility
- Internal scarring of ovaries and fallopian tubes
- Lesions and adhesions
- Abscess or rapture of ovaries
- Pelvic cysts
- Ureter and bowel blockage due to adhesions

If you have been diagnosed with endometriosis, you may wonder what to do next especially if you have chronic pelvic pain that prevents you from enjoying your life. Fortunately, there is the endometriosis diet that you can follow coupled with exercise to heal naturally.

Diet and nutrition are known to control the symptoms of endometriosis. Women who have taken the dietary approach have reported improvement in the condition and their overall health. Why don't you try it? We will offer you guidance and support throughout this book that will help you overcome the signs and symptoms which are associated with endometriosis until you regain your vibrant health again. I am sure you like that, so, keep reading.

Nutritional therapy is an important factor in dealing with this disease effectively and those who have adopted it are happy that they did. The stories of success are so motivating. When diet and nutrition are combined with regular exercise, they can control the signs and symptoms of endometriosis entirely.

You may not have endometriosis still, what we have described in this book when applied, will help you prevent suffering from it at an early age. Applying the recommendations in this book will help you combat the disease that has afflicted many women in America and all over the world.

In some people, pain is so intense while others who have the same disease may not experience any symptoms at all. That is why you should start adopting a healthy lifestyle as early as possible because some women suffer from this disease for many years without knowing it.

The effects of changing your diet

If you have been diagnosed with endometriosis, don't suffer quietly. The best thing for you is to take a healthy diet based on natural products and exercise regularly. Changing your lifestyle and diet involves making adjustments to what you consume if you have to control the symptoms.

When you change your diet you will

- Lower or eliminate the intake of toxins caused by additives, preservatives, foods affected by pesticides, herbicides, antibiotics and other chemicals given to animals like chicken.
- Reduce pain, inflammation and cramps
- Reduce constipation and bloating
- Lower estrogen levels in the body

- Modulate the hormones
- Boost your immunity to help your body fight illnesses and diseases
- Control weight if weight-loss is among your concerns

Each of these effects lower the signs and symptoms of endometriosis eliminating them entirely with time and you can enjoy what you love most as you become healthier again. Endometriosis is both a hormonal and immune system condition. That is why you need to take a diet that boosts the immune system and also modulates estrogen levels in the body.

To notice a change in endometriosis symptoms, you need to change your diet and eat healthy foods. Many of these foods like ginger and turmeric may just be right there on your kitchen shelf or cupboard. Take fresh produce, fruits and vegetables especially leafy green vegetables. Eat raw fruits and vegetables, prepare green salads, blend them or cook them lightly, in order to get all the nutrients your body needs.

Who doesn't enjoy eating those fresh fruits in season? I am sure you do. Make fruits and vegetables the main part of your diet and you will find that your vitality is back within no time.

Whenever it is possible buy organically-grown foods. This may sound difficult at the beginning but when you start feeling better you will get motivated.

You will need to start taking certain foods and avoid taking others. When you eat a healthy diet, you boost your immune system to enable it to fight diseases. That is why having a vibrant and strong immunity is the key to healing endometriosis. A change in diet boosts your energy levels improving your overall physical health.

Conventional medicine and surgery have been used for many years to treat endometriosis but eating a natural healthy diet is an effective way of reducing the symptoms of the disease and healing naturally. Our bodies respond to what we eat and how we exercise, making us healthier. If you want to stay healthy, you have to observe safe eating habits and ensure that you exercise regularly.

There are some foods that worsen the symptoms of endometriosis due to the chemical reactions they cause in the body and you should avoid them completely. Stick to the non-inflammatory diet stated in this book and you will thank yourself that you did.

When you have high levels of estrogen in your system, it causes growth of the endometrial tissue in the external surface just the same way it does in the lining of the uterus. This works naturally within the uterus but when it happens outside the uterus, the pain becomes severe, there is excessive bleeding and damage to organs such as the bowel and bladder as well as scarring in other areas like the ovaries and fallopian tubes.

Infertility can occur or you may have difficulty conceiving. That is why you should take endometriosis diet even if you have not been diagnosed with the disease. Conventional treatment includes medications and surgery to remove the endometrial tissue. However, experts have proved that diet and nutrition coupled with exercise can help to control the symptoms of endometriosis just like they do with symptoms of other estrogen related conditions like menstruation, menopause and fibroids.

2: Signs and Symptoms and How to Control Them

No matter what age you may be, your health is very important to you and your loved ones. Illnesses and diseases affect your overall health as well as your quality of life. That is why you should take charge of your health as early as possible. If you have any of the signs and symptoms associated with endometriosis, you should not worry because you can put an end to your suffering with nutritional therapy and exercise.

Signs and Symptoms

When someone has endometriosis, the tissue that in normal circumstances lines the uterus develops outside the uterus. The tissue grows on the membrane that lines the abdominal cavity and elsewhere.

The most common signs and symptoms caused by endometriosis are:

- Painful monthly periods
- Heavy periods
- Muscle cramps
- Pre-menstrual stress PMS and discomfort

- Chronic pelvic pains-acute pain in ovaries, fallopian tubes, bladder, rectum and lower abdomen due to scarring and shedding of endometrial tissue
- Lower back pain
- Irregular periods
- Spotting or excessive bleeding between periods
- Pain when urinating or with bowel movements
- Bloating and constipation
- Infertility or difficulty in getting pregnant
- Rupturing of the ovaries in extreme cases which may cause internal bleeding

You may experience discomfort in the pelvis before your menstruation especially between ovulation and the onset of monthly periods. Pre-menstrual stress PMS and discomfort is a troubling condition that many women and girls of reproductive age are concerned about. Symptoms of endometriosis may be severe in some people and may worsen over time while other endometriosis sufferers may have no symptoms at all.

Pain Stages

The pain of endometriosis ranges from minimal pain to severe pain. Yet, there are many people who suffer from this condition who report no pain. The physical disease is divided into four stages.

- Stage I is minimal pain
- Stage II is mild pain
- Stage III is moderate pain
- Stage IV is severe pain

This does not indicate the intensity of pain. Some people in the minor stage may have intense pain while someone in stage IV may have mild pain or no pain at all.

Diagnosis of endometriosis that is not physically visible is done using laparoscopy. This is a procedure that uses a camera that is inserted into the abdomen through small incisions. Biopsy is also used to diagnose the disease. Surgery is invasive, but it is the only definite method for diagnosing endometriosis.

Controlling the Signs and Symptoms of Endometriosis

The following are effective methods used in controlling and eliminating the signs and symptoms of endometriosis. Choose natural healthy methods that work without subjecting you to side effects and other complications. These are:

- Diet and nutrition
- Exercise
- Medications
- Hormonal treatments
- Surgery

Diet and nutrition

Endometriosis diet is the sure way to control the signs and symptoms of this disease. The diet does not cause any side effects like other conventional treatments. It also boosts your overall health raising your energy levels and making you vibrant again. The diet also helps you to fight other illnesses and diseases.

When endometriosis diet is combined with natural treatments it effectively combats the signs and symptoms of endometriosis and other conditions. It reduces pains, inflammation and cramps. The diet consists of foods and drinks that are full of flavor consisting of main dishes, soups, sauces, baked products, sweets, dressings, dips and spreads.

The fact that you have endometriosis or you are preventing it does not mean that you will be tied to a dull diet. No, on the contrary, you will have interesting food combinations that you will enjoy some of which are mouth-watering.

Exercise

Physical activity stimulates production of natural endorphins which relieve pain, reduce stress and fight depression. Intense exercises like running and cycling make the body to release endorphins. Go to the gym and work on different types of aerobics. Many prolonged and continuous exercises help to release high levels of endorphins to lessen pain and stress as well as to give us that feeling of euphoria. There are many other activities you can do before, during and after your periods (Chapter 7).

Medications

Pain management involves taking of over-the-counter OTC drugs like paracetamols and oral non-steroidal anti-inflammatory drugs NSAIDs like ibuprofen and NSAID injections. Other medications include opioids especially morphine.

Hormonal Treatments

There are several hormonal treatments which are used to treat endometriosis.

Progesterone or Progestin

Progesterone or Progestin are used to inhibit the formation of endometrium and to counteract estrogen which causes inflammatory reactions in the body. The progestin mostly used is Dienogest sold as Visanne. Menstrual flow may be reduced or eliminated for some time and reversed when it is required.

Oral contraceptive drugs

Oral contraceptive drugs are used to lower the effects of endometriosis. They work by lowering the hormones that contribute towards the development of endometriosis as well as reducing or eliminating menstruation flow giving relief to the sufferer. They are used as a long-term treatment to control bleeding and the duration of monthly periods. Danazol and gestrinone may also be used. Oral contraception pill OCP is used to relieve symptoms of endometriosis but it may not be good for those who want to conceive. Furthermore, some women react negatively and some of them cannot tolerate it.

Anti-gonadotropin drugs

Anti-gonadotropin drugs are used to combat the production of hormones in the ovaries where they are mainly formed. This results in lower estrogen levels and reduction of endometrial tissue. However, the drugs cause unpleasant side effects such as hot flashes due to early menopause triggered by these drugs and may eventually lead to osteoporosis.

Aromatase inhibitors

Aromatase inhibitors are another option for treating endometriosis which should be considered by those who opt for conventional treatments.

Chinese Medical Therapy

The Chinese have for centuries produced Traditional Chinese Medicines TCM based on herbs that have been used for centuries to combat illnesses and diseases with great success. Acupuncture and acupressure may also be used.

Surgery

- ### *Laparoscopy*

    Laparoscopy involves removal of endometriosis tissue through small incisions where the instruments are inserted. This procedure is used to control pelvic pain and improve fertility. Since it does not remove the uterus and ovaries then the patient has a chance to get pregnant. The advantage of laparoscopy is that the patient heals quickly and there is little scarring. However, there may be recurrence of the condition in some women.

- ***Hysterectomy***

    Hysterectomy in the most extreme cases where the patient has acute pain, excessive bleeding and cancer, hysterectomy is performed whereby the uterus and at times the ovaries are removed. Doctors recommend this procedure to women who don't wish to conceive as a last resort when other methods have failed. This is an irreversible method. When the endometriosis affects the ovaries, the patient may have acute pain and in the most severe cases, the ovaries may rupture causing internal bleeding. The lesions and adhesions in the ovaries should be removed by open surgery or laparoscopy to avoid this.

- ***Treatment of infertility***

    Treatment of infertility surgery helps in treating infertility and it is more effective than medications in this regard. The endometrial tissues are removed while the ovaries are preserved giving the woman a chance to conceive. IVFs may be used to improve fertility and assist the woman to get pregnant.

Endometriosis can persist after surgery and even after menopause. That is why taking a natural diet is important to combat any recurrence. We have seen that whether you are using medications, hormonal treatments or surgery there is no guarantee that these therapies will assure you of an endometriosis-free life, since there is the risk of recurrence of the condition in the future within 2-5 years.

Medications and surgery are beneficial because they are effective in controlling pain but recurrence of pain is high even after using either medicinal or surgical interventions. Both have advantages and disadvantages which should be considered.

The Medications taken are strong pain relievers and the treatment can be varied from time to time, and the cost is usually low. However, they are less effective when infertility is concerned, they create adverse effects such as side-effects making their usage limited over prolonged periods of time and the cost can rise when the patient is dependent on these drugs.

Surgery is effective in controlling pelvic pain and improving the chances of pregnancy in infertility, it is less invasive when laparoscopic procedure is used and it reduces the risk of post-operative adhesions making re-operative surgery possible. Laser surgery is effective but its downside is that, it leads to scarring of internal scar tissue and development of adhesions. Adhesions are fibrous bands that connect tissues after surgery (which should not be connected) and may discourage conception and cause inflammation.

However, the cost of surgery is high and it does not guarantee that the patient will not have a recurrence of endometriosis. Some procedures also cause irreversible effects like the removal of the uterus, ovaries and fallopian tubes. You therefore need to consider each option before making your choices on which therapy to opt for.

The side-effects of these treatments include formation of adhesions, artificial menopause and hot flashes associated with it, scarring when surgery is used and other adverse effects. This should bring you to the consideration of the endometriosis diet that will heal you naturally. This has no side-effects.

3: Nutritional Therapy for Treating Endometriosis

Endometriosis diet is therapeutic, curative and preventative. Treatment of endometriosis stated in this book involves pain relief, treatment of infertility, combating progression of the condition and helping women and girls to regain their health again. It helps them to understand about how their bodies work and what they can do.

Although there are many theories about what causes endometriosis, what we know is that, we can control it to our advantage because we know how the condition behaves and what we can do or not do to live a better life. We cannot allow endometriosis to control our lives. No, we can put it under control and heal naturally with the Endometriosis diet but first we need to understand what happens to our bodies so we can take charge of our lives.

Nutritional therapy uses Endometriosis diet without using drugs or surgery. Normally, what happens is that, the tissue in the uterus which is known as endometrium thickens every month in readiness to receive a fertilized egg and bear it through pregnancy.

When this does not happen because the egg (ova) has not been fertilized by the sperm, the endometrium is shed off and this is the monthly period or menstruation which causes bleeding. This is a healthy process which happens to women normally and you should not worry about it unless it is accompanied by signs and symptoms that are not usual, like excessive bleeding and irregularity. The menstrual cycle is controlled by hormones known as estrogens.

But, there are times when hormonal imbalances cause abnormal growth of endometrial tissue in other areas like in the ovaries, fallopian tubes, intestines and bladder or elsewhere as we have seen earlier in Chapter 1.

The same hormones that cause endometrium to be shed off, also cause the abnormal endometrial tissue to be shed off either during the monthly periods or at other times. This intensifies the pelvic pain which can become chronic. It also aggravates other symptoms during the periods and during these other times. Any control of these hormonal changes can be done with diet and exercise.

It is interesting that, there are women who have endometriosis who have no pain while there are others who have chronic pelvic pain who have no endometriosis. That is why proper diagnosis has to be done especially when you opt for conventional medications and treatments. So, don't start panicking if you have pain in your pelvis or other areas mentioned in this book. You should also not relax if you have no pain. That is not a guarantee that you don't have the disease.

The most troubling thing is that, although some cases are diagnosed by the doctor using physical examinations, health history of the patient, ultrasound and laparoscopy, many cases go unnoticed. What am I saying? Surgery is the only way many endometriosis cases are diagnosed and the most definite. That is why a nutritional therapy is the best news for any woman suffering from endometriosis because it is non-invasive.

Furthermore, eating the healthy endometriosis diet is safe and you don't have to worry if you have the disease or not because it is good for your overall health. Women who are in their reproductive stage who have been diagnosed with endometriosis need nutritional therapy to combat the disease and limit its progression. Women who have natural or artificial menopause are less likely to suffer from this condition, although there are some cases reported after menopause.

What have emotions got to do with endometriosis?

Emotional issues can be a contributing factor towards the development of endometriosis and many other conditions. Eating a healthy diet and exercising, uplift your moods and trigger the "feel-good" hormones. Eating avocadoes for example, fight the bad saturated fats in the body which cause inflammatory reactions which cause many illnesses and diseases.

Exercising stimulates the nervous system to produce endorphins which fight stress, depression and fatigue. Staying emotionally healthy is an advantage while preventing or fighting any of these conditions.

Adopting a Nutritional Approach

You should adopt a nutritional approach since there are many things you can prevent while you are on it. Firstly, estrogen stimulates the creation of reproduction cells among other functions, but, when it is excessive in the body it leads to abnormal growth of endometrial tissue.

Secondly, there are compounds in the environment known as xenoestrogens that behave like estrogen in our bodies which we can control using a natural healthy diet.

Thirdly, dioxins which are in the environment are known to cause endometriosis. You should not be scared if you have endometriosis because you can have control of some of these factors making your condition to improve.

Xenoestrogens and dioxins are found in meat and dairy products, plastics heated in microwaves, agricultural herbicides and pesticides all of which we can avoid. Excess estrogen can be discouraged when you consume an anti-inflammatory diet. There are many varieties of foods that are recommended.

The nutritional therapy includes:

- Eating an anti-inflammatory diet
- Taking hormone-free meat
- Eliminating dairy products in your diet
- Eating organically grown foods when it is possible
- Consuming a well-balanced diet
- Drinking plenty of pure drinking water throughout the day

Eating an anti-inflammatory diet

Non-steroidal anti-inflammatory drugs NSAIDs and injections are used in the management of endometriosis. In the same way an anti-inflammatory diet and nutrition is effective in combating the effects of endometriosis.

However, the non-steroidal anti-inflammatory drugs and injections contain chemicals since they are synthesized in their production. Eating an anti-inflammatory diet consisting of natural foods will work in the same way as NSAIDs without adding toxins to your system. An anti-inflammatory diet promotes hormonal balance and as a result, symptoms are reduced. It also controls allergies to some foods and Candida (yeast) experienced by some endometriosis sufferers.

Ginger, cinnamon and turmeric are important anti-inflammatory products. Take them fresh or ground. Add basil, thyme, rosemary, parsley and other spices and herbs in your food.

Consuming non-hormonal meats and milk

Hormonal treatments in animal husbandry contain estrogen. Eating meat and milk from these animals exposes you to additional estrogen-like chemicals which you should avoid to combat symptoms of endometriosis.

Eat only meats from animals that are not treated with hormones and avoid red meat. Eat fish instead of meat and ham. Buy salmon, mackerel, herring, sardines and other types of cold-water or deep sea fish. A better source would be organic products, like chicken and eggs.

Eliminating dairy products in your diet

Avoid consuming meat, cream, cheese, butter, whey, milk protein and cow milk, casein and other dairy products. Dairy products increase the negative prostaglandins which activate inflammation, so, if you can, avoid them or minimize their intake. Take calcium and Vitamin D supplements, nuts and seeds.

Eating organically grown foods when it is possible

You should feed your cells with natural healthy whole foods which are organically-grown. You may find them expensive but if you think of the cost incurred in treating diseases and loss of quality of life, then you will be motivated to eat healthy foods, however expensive they may be. After all, how much money do you spend on your hair, car, furniture and vacations? Your health is more important because if diseases strike, they can prevent you from enjoying these things. Invest in your health you will not regret it.

Consuming a well-balanced diet

You should eat a balanced diet if you want to fight endometriosis or any other illnesses and diseases. A whole food diet consisting of whole carbohydrates, healthy fats, proteins, plenty of fruits and vegetables, vitamins and minerals, dietary supplements, nuts and seeds which are recommended to fight endometriosis and for your overall health. A diet based on plants is better than a meat-based diet.

Drinking plenty of pure drinking water throughout the day

Drink plenty of pure water or mineral water about 8 glasses a day. You can buy bottled water or purified water and take it throughout the day. Use a water purifier to get rid of toxins in tap water that contains chlorine or if it is contaminated.

Start by eating most of dark green leafy vegetables like spinach, cruciferous vegetables like broccoli and cabbage, fruits and pumpkin seeds.
To strengthen the immune system, eat:

- Carrots which are rich in Vitamin A and beta-carotene antioxidants
- Beans, peas and lentils
- Ginger an anti-inflammatory agent
- Garlic whether raw or partially cooked
- Yogurt to add good bacteria to the intestinal tract
- Onions

- Green tea which is beneficial in many ways including eliminating dioxin acid from the system
- Seeds whether in whole or as sprouted since they are rich in nutrients
- Rhubarb

Antioxidants found in carrots, capsicum, watermelon, spinach, berries and other colored fruits and vegetables fight free radicals that cause many diseases including cancer. Endometriosis can cause cancer in severe cases.

Hormonal balancing foods

These foods contain natural plant sterols which blocks estrogen receptors in the body. They consist of phyto-estrogens which ensure that any excess estrogen in the body does not cling onto the receptors. They should however be taken in moderation to balance the hormones. Moderating estrogen in the body is very important.

- Apples
- Beans
- Berries
- Cabbage
- Carrots
- Cauliflower

- Celery
- Garlic
- Nuts like Walnuts
- Parsley
- Peas
- Pulses
- Rhubarb
- Seeds

If you take the diet recommended in this book and your symptoms still persist, don't give up because you will still be healthy in other areas.

Women who take endometriosis diet as stated in this book report improvement. There is therefore a strong relationship between diet and the disease. When you follow this practical nutritional therapy, the endometriosis will start diminishing with time.

4: Foods You Should Take

When you need to change your lifestyle and eating habits, you may ask "What is there left for me to eat?" There is a wide variety of every type of food that will make your life exciting.

Experimenting with different recipes leaves you with an urge to discover more and more food possibilities. Begin by eating a natural healthy diet and when you start feeling better no one else except you will know that following the right path of the foods you should take is so beneficial. After some time others around you especially your family and friends or colleagues will notice the change and start complimenting you because good health shows on the outside.

To regenerate your health, you need to eat fresh produce, fruits and vegetables as much as possible. They are available in many places like in grocery stores, farmers' markets, flea markets, co-operatives and elsewhere. Fruits and vegetables should be eaten raw or partially cooked for you to be able to get optimal nutritional value from them. Many nutrients like vitamins are destroyed while cooking.

As I have said earlier, eat organic foods whenever it is possible for you. They may be more expensive than processed foods but when you think about it, treating diseases is more expensive. There are organically grown produce, fruits and vegetables in the market, free range chicken and eggs available in many places. You can grow herbs and spices in pots, containers and in the garden.

There are many studies that have been conducted with results that show that, you are what you eat. Although we cannot rule out genetics and environmental influences, eating the right diet has a direct influence on your health. You need to take care of your body by taking a natural healthy diet to inhibit development and progression of endometriosis and other conditions. Eat foods that alleviate the symptoms and avoid those that aggravate it.

Carbohydrates

Take less-processed less-refined foods to get optimum nutrients from them. Eat complex starchy foods instead of the simple starches.
These include and are not limited to:

- Whole grains
- Brown rice
- Sweet potatoes
- Arrowroots
- Winter squashes
- Beans and legumes among others.

The whole grains can be eaten as a whole or crushed with the bran and the whole grain intact. Consumption of wheat and wheat products should be avoided or minimized. Eat less of wheat flour products if you cannot avoid them entirely. Wheat flour products include bread, cakes, scones, pasta and packaged snacks with wheat as one of the ingredients.

Proteins

Your consumption of proteins per day should range from 80 to 120 grams daily per 2000 calories consumed daily. Take more vegetable based proteins rather than animal based proteins. Vegetable proteins include beans and lentils among others. Eat nuts such as almonds and walnuts. You can also eat animal based proteins such as fish, natural yogurt and cheese and free-range chicken without the skin.

Fats

Saturated fats are not good for you especially if you have endometriosis, cardiovascular diseases, arthritis, obesity or diabetes.

Take healthy fats like:

- Omega 3 essential fatty acids
- Evening Primrose Oil
- Flaxseed

- Avocadoes
- Cook with extra-virgin olive oil

Fat cells in the body act as hormone storage and excess hormones stimulate inflammation. If you are overweight, you should try to lose weight.

Fruits and Vegetables

Fruits and vegetables are rich in carotenoids and flavonoids which have anti-inflammatory and anti-oxidant activities. Eat plenty of fruits and vegetables especially when they are in season. Eat them raw, blended or lightly cooked. Avoid over-cooking the food, steam the vegetables in low heat or eat them raw to get the nutrients intact.

Vegetables: Take 4-5 servings a day of raw or lightly cooked vegetables including:

- Dark green leafy vegetables-spinach, kale, collard greens, Swiss chard and others.
- Cruciferous vegetables-carrots, cabbage, cauliflower, broccoli, beets, peas, onions, Brussels sprouts, squashes among others.

Fruits: Take 2-4 servings a day of fresh, frozen or dried fruits. Choose fresh fruits which are in season or frozen fruits. These include:

- Apples

- Raspberries, strawberries, blueberries and blackberries
- Oranges
- Red grapes
- Pink grapefruits
- Peaches
- Cherries
- Pears
- Guavas
- Mangoes
- Plums
- Watermelon
- Ripe bananas among many others

Vitamins and Minerals

To get the optimal amounts of vitamins and minerals, you need to eat plenty of fresh fruits and vegetables. Choose fruits and vegetables from a wide spectrum of all of nature's colors red, green, blue, purple, black and yellow among many others which are rich in alpha and beta carotenes. These include apples, carrots, green and purple cabbage, broccoli, celery, rhubarb, spinach, tomatoes, avocado, watermelon, green, blue and yellow capsicums, strawberries, blueberries, red berries, raspberries, oranges, mangoes and others.

You should also add the following antioxidants in your diet

- *Vitamin C -* Take 200-500 mg daily
- *Mixed carotenoids and flavonoids*
- *B-complex vitamins*
- *Vitamin E - Daily intake of 400 IU mixed tocopherols*
- *Vitamin D -* This is an essential vitamin that should be taken with calcium and magnesium supplements for improved absorption of nutrients.
- *Selenium -* Daily intake of 200 micrograms of organic selenium helps fight endometriosis and cancer.

Combination of these vitamins is a good foundation that helps your metabolism to produce white blood cells which fight illnesses and diseases and act as the body's defensive mechanism. B1 and B6 vitamins help to regulate the hormones. Modulation of estrogen is vital for control of endometriosis.

Herbs and Spices

Ginger and turmeric are important anti-inflammatory products as well as cinnamon. Take them fresh as part of the ingredients in your food or ground them and add to your food or make herbal tea. Add basil, thyme, rosemary and other spices of your choice.

Nuts and Seeds

Nuts and seeds are a good source of protein, healthy fats, vitamins and minerals. Limit usage of saturated fats and oils because they contain negative prostaglandins which aggravate inflammatory reactions in the body. Use more of Omega 3 fatty oils in addition to:

- Walnuts
- Almonds
- Flaxseed
- Pumpkin seeds

Teas

Green tea is good. Drink 2-4 cups of green tea or white tea daily. When you have cramps, drink 1-2 cups of red raspberry leafy tea daily to help relieve these troubling cramps.

Fiber

Fiber intake promotes digestion reducing bloating and constipation which are some of the symptoms reported by endometriosis sufferers. Take estrogen promoting dark green vegetables which include broccoli, cabbage, mustard seeds and others.

Fiber intake includes:

- Whole grains like beans with the bran intact (wheat and wheat flour products being an exemption)
- Vegetables and fruits like beans, peas, berries and pulse
- Brown rice
- Oatmeal
- Almonds

Try to consume 40 grams of fiber daily. Eat foods that are high in natural fiber which include beans, peas, berries, whole grains like brown rice and a variety of other fruits and vegetables. Bran like rice bran is a good source of fiber but take plenty of water with it to speed up digestion.

Omega 3 Essential Fatty Oils

Oily fish and fish oils supplements, walnuts and dark green vegetables contain Omega 3 essential fatty oils. Eat oily fish like salmon, tuna, sardines, mackerel and herring. Take Omega 3 fatty acid supplements either as liquid oil or capsules. Take 1 gram a day and keep increasing your intake until you are able to take 3-4 grams a day.

Water

Drink plenty of pure drinking water every day. Our bodies consist mostly of water and without it our cells and the digestive system would create other problems.

Why You Should Take Vitamins and Minerals

B Vitamins

B vitamins help to produce the white blood cells which the body uses to fight diseases and infections. B vitamins also help in breaking down carbohydrates, proteins and fats in the system. When someone with endometriosis takes foods rich in B vitamins, they elevate their moods reducing the negative emotional symptoms associated with the disease.

Calcium

Calcium, magnesium and Vitamin D should be consumed together for improved absorption. You should take 500-700 mg calcium dietary supplements daily in addition to intake of foods rich in calcium, such as calcium citrate.

A few days before the monthly periods, the calcium in the body decreases and this causes cramps, discomfort, pelvic pain or headaches during menstruating time. Calcium intake should be increased 10 to 14 days before the onset of monthly periods. There are many sources of calcium but you can also take calcium supplements to boost the calcium levels.

Magnesium

Magnesium helps in the absorption of calcium in the body. It also aids in easing muscle cramps experienced during menstruation. It maintains the right water level in the gut controlling constipation as a result.

Vitamin A

Carrots are rich in Vitamin A which is a strong antioxidant and an immune system booster.

Vitamin C

Ascorbic acid also known as Vitamin C is popularly known to fight diseases and infections in the body. It is an effective antioxidant. Vitamin C is not stored in the body so it should be taken daily. Most fresh fruits and vegetables like oranges contain Vitamin C.

Vitamin D

This vitamin when taken with calcium strengthens bones and teeth as well as lessening discomforts like menstrual cramps.

Vitamin E

Vitamin E is an immunity booster.

Iron

Most women who have endometriosis bleed excessively during monthly periods and between periods. They therefore tend to have iron deficiency, which may lead to low hemoglobin in the blood indicating that you may have anemia. If you feel dizzy, fatigued or weak, check up with your doctor. Iron is important for women and girls who are in their reproductive stage especially if they have endometriosis. If you are one of them, you should take foods rich in iron and iron dietary supplements to replace the blood lost.

Selenium

Selenium boosts the immune system and it reduces the inflammatory symptoms commonly linked with endometriosis, especially when taken with Vitamin E.

Zinc

Zinc found in beans, peas and lentils is helpful in boosting the immune system helping the body to heal itself as a result. Many enzymes, good bacteria and vitamins are produced in the intestinal tract. When the digestive system functions as it should, the immune system is strengthened and your body is able to fight diseases like endometriosis and others. A healthy digestive system is therefore crucial in fighting endometriosis. For optimal uptake of nutrients and effective transportation of the nutrients to the organs and other parts of the body you need to eat a healthy diet.

5: Foods That You Should Avoid

Wrong food choices expose us to toxins, impurities and environmental exposures which reveal themselves as illnesses and diseases. When we consume certain foods, they wreck havoc in our systems and interfere with metabolism. These foods trigger negative immune system and hormonal reactions that cause inflammation. That is why a natural healthy diet and nutrition is a sure way to heal many illnesses and diseases including endometriosis.

Eating foods loaded with additives, preservatives, inflammatory-induced hormones and dioxins only creates a bad foundation of our health. Read the labels carefully before you buy products. However, some of the information may not be revealed on some products so it is important to use your own judgment and make informed decisions after reading this book.

Foods are also related to other conditions like gluten-intolerance, allergies and other complications.

For some people avoiding wheat products, eggs, dairy products, refined sugar, lactose, soya and soya products, refined carbohydrates, red meat, caffeine and alcohol is the sure way to go. Those with gluten-intolerance should avoid products containing gluten. Some people prefer to eat vegan foods avoiding animal proteins altogether.

Foods with additives and preservatives

Many processed foods you find on the shelves in convenience stores are loaded with additives and preservatives. They have little or no nutritional value. Read the labels before you buy your groceries. Buy fresh produce, fruits and vegetables that have been grown organically to get optimal nutritional value if you have endometriosis. If you can, grow some of the foods yourself.

The toxins in additives and preservatives overload your system and slow metabolism. The body uses a lot of energy to rid itself of these toxins, which should have been used to fight diseases and infections.

The liver breaks down estrogen and fats, so balancing hormones in your body and reducing storage of fats in the body helps the liver to perform other functions for healthy metabolism. Minimize consumption of processed foods as much as possible. Avoid fast foods and eat home cooked foods which contain all the nutrients the body needs, to stay healthy and fight illnesses and diseases.

Wheat

Wheat contains acid which is known to aggravate the symptoms of endometriosis in some women. You should therefore avoid taking wheat products that include bread, pasta products, cakes and other foods. Wheat contains gluten and most people with endometriosis report sensitivity to gluten so it is good to be on the safe side by eliminating wheat products in your diet.

Red meat

Animal proteins especially red meat promotes aggravation of bad prostaglandins and growth of hormones which cause inflammation reactions in the body causing pain and discomfort. Eat fish, nuts, legumes, nuts and seeds.

Dairy products

Avoid taking meat, cream, cheese, butter, whey, milk protein, casein and other dairy products. These products increase the negative prostaglandins which activate inflammation. When you are shopping, read the labels carefully and avoid buying products that contain these products because they contain estrogenic hormones whether in their natural form or they are artificial. None of them is good for you if you suffer from endometriosis.

Saturated fats

Saturated fats should be avoided or minimized. Take Omega 3 essential fatty oils, flaxseed oil and eat avocadoes. Avocadoes contain the good fats that fight the bad fats in the body. Use extra-virgin olive oil for cooking.

Refined sugar

Refined sugar promotes inflammation. Avoid taking sugar, honey, chocolate and foods prepared using these products.

Soy and Soy Products

Soy and soy products are rich in phytoestrogens and their intake increases estrogen levels in the body. They should therefore be avoided by women with endometriosis.

Refined carbohydrates

Refined starch should be substituted with complex carbohydrates. To lose weight, eat low-carb diets. Take complex carbohydrates like whole grains (except wheat and wheat products), brown rice, sweet potatoes, arrow roots and other carbohydrates.

Eggs

If you cannot avoid eating eggs, then buy organic ones. Most other eggs have a tendency to have dioxin chemicals that may have formed as a residue of animal husbandry treatments. Some people with endometriosis may get constipation after consuming eggs or foods prepared with eggs as one of the ingredients. Constipation worsens the symptoms.

Fructose Corn Syrup

Foods prepared with fructose corn syrup and other stabilizers should be avoided.

Hormone-induced products

Foods like meat and chicken, dairy products should be avoided. Take organically grown products when it is possible and free-range chicken (without the skin) and eggs.

Caffeine

Caffeine should be avoided.

Alcohol

Avoid taking alcohol. Alcohol interferes with the metabolism of estrogen in the system. This leads to accumulation of estrogen in the body which encourages growth of endometrial tissue.

Modulation of estrogen

Avoid foods that have xenoestrogens which have the same effect as estrogens and may lead to increased growth of endometrial tissue.

You may ask yourself if it will be possible to avoid all these foods which you have been used to for so many years. Start by introducing some of the foods you enjoy into the diet. Experiment with different recipes and see how you like them. Prepare fresh dark green vegetable as salads and cook the others lightly or eat carrots and tomatoes raw. Tell your family and friends that you plan to change your diet and lifestyle and they will help you.

6: Natural Treatments and Therapy for Healing Endometriosis

Although the causes of endometriosis are not known, there are many factors that we know can aggravate or alleviate the disease. If you have endometriosis, you may experience heavy periods and spotting or excessive bleeding in between periods, pelvic pain and infertility. That is why we have devoted this book to help you adopt effective natural therapies that heal endometriosis naturally.

Natural Treatments and Therapy

There are several successful therapies which women have sought to relief the symptoms of endometriosis, over the years.
The following are the popular natural treatments and therapies as reported by the endometriosis community, which have proved to be helpful over the years:

- Diet and Nutrition
- Exercise
- Herbal preparations
- Massage
- Weight loss
- Other Alternative Therapies and Treatments: TENS electrotherapy, Acupuncture, Shiatsu,

Biofeedback, Naturopathy, Homeopathy, Osteopathy therapies and Chiropractic

Diet and Nutrition

Some women have food intolerances that aggravate the condition and an endometriosis diet is what they need. There are people who have intolerance against gluten and avoiding wheat products like bread, pasta and cakes works well for them.

There are foods that trigger inflammatory reactions like dairy products and processed foods with additives and preservatives, so making the right choice of what to eat is important. This approach also helps the body to rid itself of toxins and impurities in the system making the digestive system able to work efficiently. A healthy digestive system is important in endometriosis cases because it is able to eliminate inflammatory foods that trigger the symptoms.

Exercise

Exercise is known to alleviate other estrogen related conditions and it is believed that it can do the same with endometriosis. Physical activity helps to create endorphins which are natural pain and stress relievers. High endorphins make us feel less pain and they reduce stress as well as fight depression. Take aerobic exercises at the gym or at home, go for jogging, cycling, hiking or taking a walk will benefit you a long way whether you have endometriosis or not.

Physical exercises that make your heart to rate faster or which make you sweat show that you are triggering the body to form endorphins. As a result, the pain you are feeling will reduce and you will start to feel better. After all who wants a painful life?

Herbal preparations

For many years, people have depended on herbal preparations for the treatment of endometriosis and many other ailments with success. Herbs and spices especially ginger and turmeric have been very successful in controlling inflammatory conditions that contributes towards the development of endometriosis.

Many herbal medicines used are prepared from roots, bark of plants, flowers, leaves and stems. The herb preparations can be ingested in tablet or capsule form or as tea, applied on the topical area, inhaled or used otherwise. Herbs can be taken as fresh or ground into a powder used in food preparation or used to prepare herbal tea. The herbs used in herbal medicine can be combined to make them more effective.

It is widely believed that herbs and spices have a major role in combating endometriosis. High levels of estrogen in the body contribute towards the signs and symptoms of this condition. One of the functions of the liver is to break down estrogen and so, when the liver is weak there is accumulation of excess estrogen in the body leading to the growth of abnormal endometrial tissue in other parts of the body other than in the uterus. Herbal treatments aimed at stimulating the liver to be able to effectively and efficiently break down estrogen to relieve the symptoms associated with this disease. The symptoms may disappear altogether after several months.

Some of the herbs used to treat pain and other symptoms are Evening Primrose Oil, Peppermint, Yam, Red Raspberry, Cranberry, Blue Cohosh, Black Cohosh, Plantain, Couchgrass, Valerian White Willow and others.

However, you should note that, although herbs and spices are natural, they can also be toxic. You should therefore seek the advice of your health care provider if you want to start herbal therapy especially if you are taking other types of medications.

Traditional Chinese Medicine - TCM

Traditional Chinese Medicine uses herbal remedies and other methods. You can experiment with these types of medicines which have been used for centuries to heal many ailments. The Chinese approach aims at strengthening the immune system for body to heal illnesses and diseases and maintain health by stimulating the defense mechanism using herbal medicines, acupuncture, acupressure and other therapies.

The herbal formulas are antibacterial, antiviral and immune system boosters. They are available as pills or as tea extracts. Some herbal remedies are very effective and they are able to heal diseases that conventional treatments are unable to. They are therapeutic and can treat other conditions apart from endometriosis.

TCM is also used to treat asthma and allergies as well as to relieve dental pain, chronic low back pain, arthritis, osteoarthritis, migraine headaches, Parkinson's disease and fibromyalgia. TCM is used to deal with anxiety, post-traumatic stress disorder and depression, vomiting, nausea and irritable bowel syndrome. When used with in-vitro fertilization TCM can induce pregnancy even in sufferers of endometriosis.

In acupuncture thin needles are used while pressure of the acupuncture points is used in acupressure without the needles. The TCM practitioner will assess you thoroughly before recommending any treatment or therapy. The treatment recommended will aim at treating the whole being for overall health instead of one condition.

Massage

Most of us know the benefits associated with massage to relieve pain and other symptoms. Many women with endometriosis use massage to relax the muscle cramps and relieve pelvic pain. Some place hot water bottles on the pelvis. Massage therapy stimulates production of natural endorphins which relieve pain and decrease stress.

Weight loss

Fat cells act as storage of hormones and so, if you are obese, you may have an accumulation of excess hormones in your body. Many fat cells in your system may trigger or worsen endometriosis. Weight loss is recommended for women who have estrogen-related complications. As you lose fat weight, you start to feel better, look better and regain your health and shape.

Other Common Alternative Therapies and Treatments

Before you try any of the alternative therapies and treatments you should seek advice from your health care provider. You should also consult licensed professional practitioners who have the knowledge and experience of providing the services to be on the safe side.

TENS electrotherapy

Transcutaneous Electrical Nerve Stimulator TENS electrotherapy uses an electrical device to conduct electrodes to painful areas to relieve them of pain. The electrical current activates the nerves. This can be an effective technique which can relieve pain quickly. You can purchase a portable unit to apply when you have pain.

Acupuncture

In acupuncture, endometriosis is treated by inserting thin needles in strategic points on the skin by a professional practitioner to relieve pain, menstrual cramps, post-operative pain and other symptoms. The Chinese practicing this therapy believe that illness results from lack of balance of Chia energy. This also causes stagnation and obstruction of energy.

They therefore use the thin needles on certain points to bring balance and free flow of energy which leads to good health resulting in pain relief and elimination of other symptoms. If acupuncture is not available where you live, you can check with medical associations. Acupuncture is known to stimulate endorphin which is a natural painkiller formed in the central nervous system and in the pituitary glands.

Shiatsu

This is a finger-pressing technique used by the Japanese to release Ki for balancing free flow which as a result relieves pain. It is like what we know as massage and the practitioner might recommend some exercises which you can do at home.

Biofeedback

Biofeedback is a relaxation technique which uses electrodes that work by altering certain processes of the body.

Naturopathy

As the name indicates, naturopathy cures using nature or natural methods. Healing comes as a result of a combination of:

- vitamin and mineral therapy
- fasting
- physical exercise
- breathing exercises
- joint manipulation
- massage

- color therapy
- acupuncture
- hydrotherapy among other factors

Homeopathy

Natural remedies which are part of the disease are used to heal the disease itself.

Aromatherapy

This therapy uses aromatic plant-based oils like sage, lavender, cypress, bergamot, fennel and others which are said to have anti-bacterial, anti-viral and anti-fungal properties, to treat endometriosis.

Phytotherapy

Phytotherapy is using plants and plant extracts to control symptoms. Some people control illnesses and diseased by avoiding meat and dairy products and eating vegan diets.

Osteopathy

This method uses muscle, bone and ligament manipulation, to correct structural problems in order to relieve the body of pain and other symptoms.

Chiropractic treatment

Chiropractics use manipulation of musculoskeletal system believing that, healing can be attained by correcting the dislocations in the system which known as subluxations. This is said to strengthen immunity.

These treatments and therapies may not be embraced by everybody. Go for what works best for you. Consult a licensed health care provider to advice you. Some of these methods used may not work singly but may require a combination of several of them.

7: Exercise and Endometriosis

Experts have proven that physical activity alleviates signs and symptoms of estrogen-related conditions like menstruation, menopause and fibroids. It should therefore be the same for endometriosis signs and symptoms. Jogging, walking, running, cycling and aerobics in the gym or at home can be done. You can take up other activities like dancing and gardening which can be a lot of fun.

Endorphin

Endorphins are our natural pain relievers and our stress fighters created by the body itself. They are known as neurotransmitters because they transmit electrical pain signals in our nervous systems.

Endorphin or endogenous morphine is produced in the central nervous system and also in the pituitary gland and elsewhere within the brain. Endo means endogenous while orphin means morphine. Orphin is a body chemical that is like morphine.

That is why synthesized opioids especially morphine are made with the same qualities of the natural body morphine. Fortunately, the natural endorphins do not have side effects like dependency and addiction found in medications such as morphine and codeine, so we should depend more on them.

The main function of endorphins produced by our bodies is to inhibit pain signal transmissions and it also creates a euphoria feeling. This inhabitation of pain signal transmissions relieves pain while the euphoria feeling, fights stress and depression. That is why endorphin production plays a major role in relieving pain in endometriosis sufferers as well as uplifting the moods of sufferers who have stress and depression.

Pain, cramps and heavy bleeding can cause the woman to have stress and depression may crop in as well. Who wants to be depressed? This makes a good reason for you to leave the couch and start exercising right away.

Endorphins are known to also stimulate immune responses, modulate appetite and other positive processes for healthy metabolism so, we should stimulate their production. When we exercise, we create high endorphin levels which relief pain and overcome the effects of stress on their own. Different people create different levels of endorphins even with the same type of exercise.

You can take red peppers to stimulate the production of endorphins especially very spicy ones. Chocolate is also craved by people with stress but it is not recommended for women with endometriosis because of the refined sugar used in their preparation.

Cytokines

Physical activity when done regularly stimulates high levels of cytokines which are known to have anti-inflammatory and antioxidants. That is why regular exercise is important for people with inflammatory diseases. Antioxidants also prevent the body from free radicals that cause illnesses and diseases. Exercise is therefore vital and should be done regularly.

What you should know about endometriosis

Every woman needs to know about endometriosis whether she has been diagnosed with it or not. This will help her to take measures as stated in this book to prevent the condition as early as possible and to remain healthy. It will help her be able to deal with it in case she is diagnosed with it. Many women and girls suffer quietly but that is because they do not know that they can get relief without incurring high initial costs. Jogging, running and walking are some of the things you can do without having to pay a single coin.

The most common signs and symptoms caused by endometriosis are:

- Painful monthly periods-exercise as much as possible. If you are unable to do any exercises during your periods because of pain, cramps and bleeding, do vigorous exercises for about 2 hours a day before the periods start.
- Pelvic pains-there are several exercises you can do even when you are sitting, standing or lying down.
- Pain in ovaries, fallopian tubes, bladder, rectum and abdomen due to scarring caused by endometrial tissues can cause stress which can be alleviated with endorphins during exercise.
- Excessive bleeding-take foods rich in iron or take iron dietary supplements.
- Pain when urinating and passing bowels-try pelvic and bowel exercises.
- Infertility or difficulty becoming pregnant-in-vitro fertilization may be used in combination with therapy. Exercise doesn't interfere with fertility.
- Bleeding between menstrual periods-exercise regularly.

Symptoms may be severe in some people and increase over time while pain and cramps can be alleviated with exercise.

The advantages of physical activity include:

- Minimal cost
- Flexibility of modifying physical therapy to what works best for you
- No major side-effects
- Triggering production of endorphins
- No interference with fertility

Physical therapy may not work on its own but may need to be combined with the endometriosis diet for it to be effective.

Relationship between Physical Activity and Endorphin

Physical activity is known to stimulate the production of natural endorphin in the body. Intense exercises that make you to breathe harder and make the heart to rate faster make the body to release endorphins to the painful parts of the body. That is why it is vital for you to engage in physical activity if you have endometriosis and even if you don't have it. Take up a gym class and work on aerobics and weight-lifting to relief pain and fight stress and depression.

We should do prolonged and continuous exercises for our bodies to release high levels of endorphins to make our pain and stress less and make us feel good due to the euphoria. Although you may not get involved in vigorous athletic activities, there are many other activities you can do before, during and after you experience the symptoms of endometriosis.

Exercises you can do

Women and girls who exercise regularly report improvement in endometriosis symptoms. However, everyone is different so, if you have worsened symptoms when you exercise follow a mild exercising approach or relax for some time until you feel better.

Breathing exercises

When you wake up in the morning, stretch yourself and do breathing exercises to start off your day. Deep breathing exercises involve inhaling deeply through the nose, holding and exhaling through the mouth. This releases carbon dioxide trapped in your system and allows oxygenated blood to flow into the cells in your body. Oxygen in the cells releases stress in the metabolism lowering stress and pain in the body. Repeat breathing exercises several times with the windows open to let in fresh air if you are exercising indoors.

Aerobics

Register in a gym class and follow an exercise regimen that works best for you. Increase speed and intensity progressively every week. Give yourself time to relax so you do not get burn out.

Walking

Walking briskly for about 30 minutes every morning, lunch time or evening is something anyone can do and it is costless. This allows blood to flow to the whole body especially to the pelvis to reduce inflammatory stress. If you stay near your workplace or college, walk on some days instead of driving. If you are driving, park in the farthest part at the parking lot and walk. Walk up and down the stairs instead of taking the elevator.

Jogging

Jogging is costless and you can jog around your surroundings either alone or with a group of neighbors.

Running

Running is known to lower estrogen levels which in turn reduce pelvic inflammation. Medium to high intensity running can control the debilitating symptoms to some extent.

Cycling

Cycling with a stationary cycle or a moving bicycle is something you can enjoy. Learn to mountain-bike. Ride a bicycle when going to college or to work instead of driving but ensure that you are safe by observing traffic road signs. Cycling is good for the cardiovascular system, joints, muscles, tendons and ligaments and for endometriosis.

Dancing

Take a ballet class or any other type of dancing that you enjoy.

Swimming

Go for swimming a few days before the onset of your monthly periods and on other days in order to relieve the symptoms of endometriosis. Swimming exercises the whole body and it is also good for those with cardiovascular problems, obesity and arthritis.

Hiking

People enjoy hiking as part of their physical activity and to see the natural scenery. Join a hiking group that visits places you would like to see.

Gardening

Grow flowers, spices and herbs in your garden, pots or containers.

Sport activities

Get yourself involve in sporting activities that you enjoy. These include women football, tennis, cricket, netball, volleyball, bowling, racing and other sports.

Physical activity has a positive impact on endometriosis and you should therefore create time every day to exercise. Make exercises your friend and enjoy them. Change your attitude to be able to embrace the benefits that come with exercises.

8: Adopt Dietary and Lifestyle Changes to Manage Endometriosis

There are many people who have allergies and food intolerances like gluten. A diet that avoids wheat and wheat products, eggs, dairy products like milk, butter and cheese, refined sugar, refined carbohydrates, lactose, soya and soya products, red meat, caffeine, alcohol and gluten would be the best to manage endometriosis. Let us first look at conventional management treatments and compare them with dietary and lifestyle changes.

Conventional Management Treatments

- Medications
- Surgery
- Hormonal therapy
- Treatment of infertility

Medications

There are different types of medications that are used to manage endometriosis. These include:

- *NSAIDs*

    Non-steroid anti-inflammatory drugs NSAIDs are used in combating the symptoms of endometriosis. These drugs may or may not be used with other types of therapy depending on the severity of the condition. NSAID injections are given when the symptoms aggravate and when oral NSAIDs interfere with stomach conditions like in people with gastro-intestinal ulcers limiting their effectiveness. That is why taking endometriosis diet is highly recommended because it has no side effects. Severe cases of endometriosis can be treated with narcotics but a natural therapy is your best option.

- ***Opioids***

These are very effective in the treatment of endometriosis especially Morphine sulphate tablets or injections. Opioids work by mimicking endorphins which are naturally occurring painkillers that are triggered in the body by physical activity. These pain reducer chemicals can be activated naturally without adding artificial chemicals into your system by following the Endometriosis diet and exercise.

- ***Other medications***

Many other medications are used but they are either less effective or they may cause adverse side effects.

Surgery

Endometriosis symptoms can become so severe that, some women opt for surgery to reduce the symptoms or give the sufferer a chance to conceive. Surgery is more of a diagnostic procedure but it can be used to treat endometriosis. The surgical procedure may involve removal of endometrial tissue known as endometrium and adhesions as well as work on the restoration of the pelvis and other parts of the body to their natural state as much as it is possible.

Some people opt for laparoscopy since it is less invasive since only very small incisions are made on the belly. The endometrium and adhesions are removed with laparoscope instruments which are inserted through the incisions. Afterwards, only small scars are left where the incisions were and the patient heals faster than if she had undergone open pelvic surgery which also causes adhesions in many women.

These adhesions can cause infertility, chronic pain in the pelvis and abdomen as well as other complications. Furthermore, when the patient needs re-operative surgery, the adhesions make it difficult. Since only the endometrial tissue is incised while the uterus and ovaries are preserved in women who wish to conceive, the condition may recur between 2 to 5 years. There is a 40-50% chance of endometriosis recurrence within 5 years when conventional surgery is used.

For women who do not wish to conceive, incision of endometriosis tissue followed by removal of the uterus may be the best option to eliminate pain and avoid the risks of recurrence. However, incision must be done otherwise pain might persist even with the removal of the uterus.
In the most severe cases, nerves to the uterus may be severed to control acute pain but this procedure is rarely used since it results in complications that are usually irreversible.

You should know that it is safe to try the endometriosis diet whether you are diagnosed with the problem or not.

Hormonal Therapy

Progesterone is a steroid hormone that inhibits the growth of endometrial tissue while it counteracts the production and circulation of estrogen in the body. Progesterone is the main steroidal hormone among the progestogens in the body that deals with formation of the embryo after fertilization, menstrual cycles and pregnancy. It also helps in the formation of other steroids in the system including corticosteroids.

Progesterone controls inflammation and regulates estrogen effects. It is produced mostly in the ovaries and to some extent in the adrenal glands and nervous tissue and also in the placenta during pregnancy but it is also synthesized. Progesterone is marketed in different trade names.

Progestin is produced to work like the natural progesterone. Dienogest is a progestin type used to treat endometriosis and sold using Visanne as the trade name.

However, taking a diet rich in all the foods stated in this book has a positive effect in healing endometriosis.

Treatment of infertility

Surgery is performed to treat infertility caused by endometriosis and it is more effective than medications. The endometrial tissues are removed while leaving the ovaries and normal tissues intact. The woman is given IVFs to encourage conception.

Management of Endometriosis using Dietary and Lifestyle Changes

There are some simple steps you should take.

- Buy colorful fruits and vegetables from a whole spectrum of colors. These will act as antioxidants and carotenoids in your diet.

- Tell your family and friends what you are doing so that they can encourage you to eat healthy. This will make you accountable.

- Wash and cut a lot of veggies and store of them in your refrigerator. Store pre-washed fruits in the refrigerator also. Instead of reaching in for a snack which is loaded with ingredients that you should avoid, open your fridge reach for fruit or vegetables. It is easier to eat them when they are already prepared than when they are not.

- Change your diet to avoid exposure to xenoestrogens. Avoid non-organic dairy products, chicken and beef which have been treated with growth hormones. Avoid foods sprayed with pesticides and herbicides or meat from animals treated with antibiotics, <u>Eliminate</u> them from your diet completely.

- Eat organic foods which do not have artificial hormones like xenoestrogens or dioxin chemical residues from pesticides. This is to avoid overloading your body with estrogen-like hormones and dioxin chemicals that contribute towards the development of endometriosis.

- Eat the endometriosis diet which is based on a well-balanced diet based on nutrient-rich foods including plenty of fresh dark green vegetables and cruciferous vegetables, fruits, cold-water fish, fiber and plenty of pure drinking water. These foods eliminate excess estrogen from the body and balance the hormones in your system so that only what is needed for healthy metabolism is maintained.
- There are many recipes online or in books that are based on a vegetable diet. You can prepare vegan foods or minimize your meat intake. Going forward, increase the dark green vegetables like spinach and kale in your meals while you minimize meat, soy and dairy products if you cannot avoid them.
- Take Omega 3 essential fatty acids supplements in liquid or oil form to fight inflammation. Eat fatty cold-water fish. Minimize the intake of saturated fats by eating plant-based foods. Eat lean white meat if you have to eat meat.
- Minimize further exposure to xenoestrogens in the environment. Don't microwave food in plastic containers or wraps. Use ceramic containers to microwave food. Don't use plastics to store food, use glass containers which are safe from xenoestrogens.

- Eat foods that are rich in vitamins and minerals especially calcium and magnesium or take supplements to recoup for any deficiencies in the diet. Eat foods with high intake of iron or take iron supplements if you bleed excessively during or between your monthly periods.
- You should take whole foods with the bran on to increase your intake of nutrients and fiber. Minimize processed food which have little nutrient value and have been loaded with refined sugars, additives and preservatives. Watch your carbohydrate intake to regulate insulin in the body. Don't overload your system with refined sugars and refined carbohydrates which interfere with metabolism of insulin pre-disposing you to diabetes. Eat proteins and low-carb diets and healthy fats to balance hormones in your body.
- Avoid saturated fats and take healthy fats which do not add excess estrogen levels to your body. Overweight women may already have excess estrogen in their systems because body fat encourages production of estrogen. Take Omega 3 fatty acids, eat avocadoes and cook with extra-virgin olive oil. Hard-pressed

- flaxseed oil is also good. You can also grind flaxseeds and add them to food ingredients.
- Phytotherapy is a diet based on plant and plant extracts. Eat vegan diets to modulate the hormones and discourage progression of endometriosis.
- Exercise with a friend. You may fail to visit the gym on some days or go for jogging when you are alone but you may not want to disappoint a friend. Take a walk in the morning or during lunch hour or any other time. Take your pet for a walk when you are at home.
- There are many activities you can do which you enjoy like gardening, cycling, swimming, taking a dance class, walking up the stairs instead of taking the elevator and others.

Conclusion

It is now clear that, what is recommended in this book will be of great help to you. Our bodies speak to us when something goes wrong and the message is loud and clear. We should listen to what our bodies tell us because if we don't, we get illnesses and diseases which may take long to heal. We all want to be healthy.

Eating the right foods and avoiding the wrong foods, as stated in this book, helps to alleviate endometriosis and other diseases. If only we can eat natural healthy foods and exercise regularly early enough, we can enjoy life and have quality of life.

It is never too late to start on the Endometriosis Diet, start now and prevent and cure endometriosis naturally. "The Endometriosis Diet: *Healing Naturally with Nutritional Therapy*" is a must-read for all women and girls who are at a risk of suffering from endometriosis.

Printed in Poland
by Amazon Fulfillment
Poland Sp. z o.o., Wrocław